This journal belongs to:

_____

My Mediterranean Diet Journal

ISBN 13: 9781793371591

Mediterranean Diet Food Shopping List

OLIVE OIL, OLIVES, VINEGARS
Extra Virgin Olive Oil
Olives
Balsamic Vinegar
Red Wine Vinegar

HERBS & SPICES
Parsley
Oregano
Basil
Dill
Thyme
Sage
Rosemary
Mint
Bay Leaves
Salt
Pepper
Cumin
Ginger
Turmeric
Saffron
Paprika
Cinnamon
Cloves
Red Pepper Flakes

GREENS
Spinach
Arugula
Lettuce
Kale
Purslane
Broccoli Rabe
Beet Greens
Collard Greens
Dandelion Greens
Mustard Greens
Turnip Greens

NUTS
Pine Nuts
Walnuts
Almonds
Chesnuts

SEEDS
Sesame Seeds
Pumpkin Seeds
Sunflower Seeds
Tahini

VEGETABLES
Onions
Garlic
Potatoes
Artichokes
Zucchini
Eggplant
Squash
Corn
Cucumbers
Broccoli
Cauliflower
Mushrooms
Beets
Carrots
Celery
Peppers
Fennel
Cabbage
Leeks

BEANS & LEGUMES
Lentils
Split Peas
Broad Beans
Chickpeas
Kidney Beans
Green Beans
Black Beans
Black Eyed Beans

WHOLE GRAINS RICE & PASTA
Whole Wheat
Bulgur Wheat
Quinoa
Rice
Orzo
Pasta
Barley

CHEESE & FERMENTED DAIRY
Feta Cheese
Mozzarella
Parmesan
Ricotta
Yogurt

FRUIT
Grapes
Tomatoes
Lemons
Oranges
Grapefruit
Apricots
Apples
Pears
Pomegranate
Cherries
Avocado
Watermelon
Honeydew
Peaches
Strawberries
Figs
Kiwi
Limes
Plums

MEAT & SEAFOOD
Chicken
Beef
Pork
Veal
Eggs
Clams
Crab
Halibut
Salmon
Sea Bass
Sardines & Anchovies
Mussels & Clams
Tuna

Date _____   Su   Mo   Tu   We   Th   Fr   Sa

Meal 1   **Time:**

Food / Beverage	Cals	Carbs	Fat	Protein
Subtotals				

Meal 2   **Time:**

Food / Beverage	Cals	Carbs	Fat	Protein
Subtotals				

Meal 3   **Time:**

Food / Beverage	Cals	Carbs	Fat	Protein
Subtotals				

8 oz. servings of water ☐ ☐ ☐ ☐ ☐ ☐ ☐ ☐

Meal 4   Time:

Food / Beverage	Cals	Carbs	Fat	Protein
Subtotals				

Meal 5   Time:

Food / Beverage	Cals	Carbs	Fat	Protein
Subtotals				

Cals	Carbs	Fat	Protein		Weight

Notes / Excercise

Date _____   Su   Mo   Tu   We   Th   Fr   Sa

Meal 1   **Time:**

Food / Beverage	Cals	Carbs	Fat	Protein
Subtotals				

Meal 2   **Time:**

Food / Beverage	Cals	Carbs	Fat	Protein
Subtotals				

Meal 3   **Time:**

Food / Beverage	Cals	Carbs	Fat	Protein
Subtotals				

8 oz. servings of water ☐ ☐ ☐ ☐ ☐ ☐ ☐ ☐

Meal 4   Time:

Food / Beverage	Cals	Carbs	Fat	Protein
Subtotals				

Meal 5   Time:

Food / Beverage	Cals	Carbs	Fat	Protein
Subtotals				

Cals	Carbs	Fat	Protein

Weight

Notes / Excercise

Date _____   Su   Mo   Tu   We   Th   Fr   Sa

Meal 1   **Time:**

Food / Beverage	Cals	Carbs	Fat	Protein
Subtotals				

Meal 2   **Time:**

Food / Beverage	Cals	Carbs	Fat	Protein
Subtotals				

Meal 3   **Time:**

Food / Beverage	Cals	Carbs	Fat	Protein
Subtotals				

8 oz. servings of water ☐ ☐ ☐ ☐ ☐ ☐ ☐ ☐

Meal 4   Time:

Food / Beverage	Cals	Carbs	Fat	Protein
Subtotals				

Meal 5   Time:

Food / Beverage	Cals	Carbs	Fat	Protein
Subtotals				

Cals	Carbs	Fat	Protein	Weight

Notes / Excercise

_____

_____

_____

Date _____   Su   Mo   Tu   We   Th   Fr   Sa

Meal 1   **Time:**

Food / Beverage	Cals	Carbs	Fat	Protein
Subtotals				

Meal 2   **Time:**

Food / Beverage	Cals	Carbs	Fat	Protein
Subtotals				

Meal 3   **Time:**

Food / Beverage	Cals	Carbs	Fat	Protein
Subtotals				

8 oz. servings of water ☐ ☐ ☐ ☐ ☐ ☐ ☐ ☐

Meal 4   Time:

Food / Beverage	Cals	Carbs	Fat	Protein
Subtotals				

Meal 5   Time:

Food / Beverage	Cals	Carbs	Fat	Protein
Subtotals				

Cals	Carbs	Fat	Protein		Weight

Notes / Excercise
_____

_____

_____

Date _____   Su   Mo   Tu   We   Th   Fr   Sa

Meal 1   **Time:**

Food / Beverage	Cals	Carbs	Fat	Protein
Subtotals				

Meal 2   **Time:**

Food / Beverage	Cals	Carbs	Fat	Protein
Subtotals				

Meal 3   **Time:**

Food / Beverage	Cals	Carbs	Fat	Protein
Subtotals				

8 oz. servings of water ☐ ☐ ☐ ☐ ☐ ☐ ☐ ☐

Meal 4   Time:

Food / Beverage	Cals	Carbs	Fat	Protein
Subtotals				

Meal 5   Time:

Food / Beverage	Cals	Carbs	Fat	Protein
Subtotals				

Cals	Carbs	Fat	Protein

Weight

Notes / Excercise

_____

_____

_____

Date _____   Su   Mo   Tu   We   Th   Fr   Sa

Meal 1   **Time:**

Food / Beverage	Cals	Carbs	Fat	Protein
Subtotals				

Meal 2   **Time:**

Food / Beverage	Cals	Carbs	Fat	Protein
Subtotals				

Meal 3   **Time:**

Food / Beverage	Cals	Carbs	Fat	Protein
Subtotals				

8 oz. servings of water ☐ ☐ ☐ ☐ ☐ ☐ ☐ ☐

Meal 4   Time:

Food / Beverage	Cals	Carbs	Fat	Protein
Subtotals				

Meal 5   Time:

Food / Beverage	Cals	Carbs	Fat	Protein
Subtotals				

Cals	Carbs	Fat	Protein	Weight

Notes / Excercise

_____

_____

_____

Date _____   Su   Mo   Tu   We   Th   Fr   Sa

Meal 1   **Time:**

Food / Beverage	Cals	Carbs	Fat	Protein
Subtotals				

Meal 2   **Time:**

Food / Beverage	Cals	Carbs	Fat	Protein
Subtotals				

Meal 3   **Time:**

Food / Beverage	Cals	Carbs	Fat	Protein
Subtotals				

8 oz. servings of water ☐ ☐ ☐ ☐ ☐ ☐ ☐ ☐

Meal 4   Time:

Food / Beverage	Cals	Carbs	Fat	Protein
Subtotals				

Meal 5   Time:

Food / Beverage	Cals	Carbs	Fat	Protein
Subtotals				

Cals	Carbs	Fat	Protein	Weight

Notes / Excercise

Date _____   Su   Mo   Tu   We   Th   Fr   Sa

Meal 1   **Time:**

Food / Beverage	Cals	Carbs	Fat	Protein
Subtotals				

Meal 2   **Time:**

Food / Beverage	Cals	Carbs	Fat	Protein
Subtotals				

Meal 3   **Time:**

Food / Beverage	Cals	Carbs	Fat	Protein
Subtotals				

8 oz. servings of water ☐ ☐ ☐ ☐ ☐ ☐ ☐ ☐

Meal 4   Time:

Food / Beverage	Cals	Carbs	Fat	Protein
Subtotals				

Meal 5   Time:

Food / Beverage	Cals	Carbs	Fat	Protein
Subtotals				

Cals	Carbs	Fat	Protein		Weight

Notes / Excercise

_____

_____

Date _____   Su   Mo   Tu   We   Th   Fr   Sa

Meal 1   **Time:**

Food / Beverage	Cals	Carbs	Fat	Protein
Subtotals				

Meal 2   **Time:**

Food / Beverage	Cals	Carbs	Fat	Protein
Subtotals				

Meal 3   **Time:**

Food / Beverage	Cals	Carbs	Fat	Protein
Subtotals				

8 oz. servings of water ☐ ☐ ☐ ☐ ☐ ☐ ☐ ☐

Meal 4   Time:

Food / Beverage	Cals	Carbs	Fat	Protein
Subtotals				

Meal 5   Time:

Food / Beverage	Cals	Carbs	Fat	Protein
Subtotals				

Cals	Carbs	Fat	Protein		Weight

Notes / Excercise

Date _____   Su   Mo   Tu   We   Th   Fr   Sa

Meal 1   **Time:**

Food / Beverage	Cals	Carbs	Fat	Protein
Subtotals				

Meal 2   **Time:**

Food / Beverage	Cals	Carbs	Fat	Protein
Subtotals				

Meal 3   **Time:**

Food / Beverage	Cals	Carbs	Fat	Protein
Subtotals				

8 oz. servings of water ☐ ☐ ☐ ☐ ☐ ☐ ☐ ☐

Meal 4   Time:

Food / Beverage	Cals	Carbs	Fat	Protein
Subtotals				

Meal 5   Time:

Food / Beverage	Cals	Carbs	Fat	Protein
Subtotals				

Cals	Carbs	Fat	Protein

Weight

Notes / Excercise

Date _____   Su   Mo   Tu   We   Th   Fr   Sa

Meal 1   **Time:**

Food / Beverage	Cals	Carbs	Fat	Protein
Subtotals				

Meal 2   **Time:**

Food / Beverage	Cals	Carbs	Fat	Protein
Subtotals				

Meal 3   **Time:**

Food / Beverage	Cals	Carbs	Fat	Protein
Subtotals				

8 oz. servings of water ☐ ☐ ☐ ☐ ☐ ☐ ☐ ☐

Meal 4   Time:

Food / Beverage	Cals	Carbs	Fat	Protein
Subtotals				

Meal 5   Time:

Food / Beverage	Cals	Carbs	Fat	Protein
Subtotals				

Cals	Carbs	Fat	Protein	Weight

Notes / Excercise

Date _____   Su   Mo   Tu   We   Th   Fr   Sa

Meal 1   **Time:**

Food / Beverage	Cals	Carbs	Fat	Protein
Subtotals				

Meal 2   **Time:**

Food / Beverage	Cals	Carbs	Fat	Protein
Subtotals				

Meal 3   **Time:**

Food / Beverage	Cals	Carbs	Fat	Protein
Subtotals				

8 oz. servings of water ☐ ☐ ☐ ☐ ☐ ☐ ☐ ☐

Meal 4   Time:

Food / Beverage	Cals	Carbs	Fat	Protein
Subtotals				

Meal 5   Time:

Food / Beverage	Cals	Carbs	Fat	Protein
Subtotals				

Cals	Carbs	Fat	Protein	Weight

Notes / Excercise

Date _____   Su   Mo   Tu   We   Th   Fr   Sa

Meal 1   **Time:**

Food / Beverage	Cals	Carbs	Fat	Protein
Subtotals				

Meal 2   **Time:**

Food / Beverage	Cals	Carbs	Fat	Protein
Subtotals				

Meal 3   **Time:**

Food / Beverage	Cals	Carbs	Fat	Protein
Subtotals				

8 oz. servings of water ☐ ☐ ☐ ☐ ☐ ☐ ☐ ☐

Meal 4   Time:

Food / Beverage	Cals	Carbs	Fat	Protein
Subtotals				

Meal 5   Time:

Food / Beverage	Cals	Carbs	Fat	Protein
Subtotals				

Cals	Carbs	Fat	Protein	Weight

Notes / Excercise

Date _____   Su   Mo   Tu   We   Th   Fr   Sa

Meal 1   **Time:**

Food / Beverage	Cals	Carbs	Fat	Protein
Subtotals				

Meal 2   **Time:**

Food / Beverage	Cals	Carbs	Fat	Protein
Subtotals				

Meal 3   **Time:**

Food / Beverage	Cals	Carbs	Fat	Protein
Subtotals				

8 oz. servings of water ☐ ☐ ☐ ☐ ☐ ☐ ☐ ☐

Meal 4   Time:

Food / Beverage	Cals	Carbs	Fat	Protein
Subtotals				

Meal 5   Time:

Food / Beverage	Cals	Carbs	Fat	Protein
Subtotals				

Cals	Carbs	Fat	Protein

Weight

Notes / Excercise
_____
_____
_____

Date _____   Su   Mo   Tu   We   Th   Fr   Sa

Meal 1   Time:

Food / Beverage	Cals	Carbs	Fat	Protein
Subtotals				

Meal 2   Time:

Food / Beverage	Cals	Carbs	Fat	Protein
Subtotals				

Meal 3   Time:

Food / Beverage	Cals	Carbs	Fat	Protein
Subtotals				

8 oz. servings of water ☐ ☐ ☐ ☐ ☐ ☐ ☐ ☐

Meal 4   Time:

Food / Beverage	Cals	Carbs	Fat	Protein
Subtotals				

Meal 5   Time:

Food / Beverage	Cals	Carbs	Fat	Protein
Subtotals				

Cals	Carbs	Fat	Protein	Weight

Notes / Excercise

Date _____   Su   Mo   Tu   We   Th   Fr   Sa

Meal 1   **Time:**

Food / Beverage	Cals	Carbs	Fat	Protein
Subtotals				

Meal 2   **Time:**

Food / Beverage	Cals	Carbs	Fat	Protein
Subtotals				

Meal 3   **Time:**

Food / Beverage	Cals	Carbs	Fat	Protein
Subtotals				

8 oz. servings of water ☐ ☐ ☐ ☐ ☐ ☐ ☐ ☐

Meal 4   Time:

Food / Beverage	Cals	Carbs	Fat	Protein
Subtotals				

Meal 5   Time:

Food / Beverage	Cals	Carbs	Fat	Protein
Subtotals				

Cals	Carbs	Fat	Protein

Weight

Notes / Excercise

Date _____   Su   Mo   Tu   We   Th   Fr   Sa

Meal 1   Time:

Food / Beverage	Cals	Carbs	Fat	Protein
Subtotals				

Meal 2   Time:

Food / Beverage	Cals	Carbs	Fat	Protein
Subtotals				

Meal 3   Time:

Food / Beverage	Cals	Carbs	Fat	Protein
Subtotals				

8 oz. servings of water ☐ ☐ ☐ ☐ ☐ ☐ ☐ ☐

Meal 4   Time:

Food / Beverage	Cals	Carbs	Fat	Protein
Subtotals				

Meal 5   Time:

Food / Beverage	Cals	Carbs	Fat	Protein
Subtotals				

Cals	Carbs	Fat	Protein

Weight

Notes / Excercise

_____

_____

_____

Date _____   Su   Mo   Tu   We   Th   Fr   Sa

Meal 1   **Time:**

Food / Beverage	Cals	Carbs	Fat	Protein
Subtotals				

Meal 2   **Time:**

Food / Beverage	Cals	Carbs	Fat	Protein
Subtotals				

Meal 3   **Time:**

Food / Beverage	Cals	Carbs	Fat	Protein
Subtotals				

8 oz. servings of water ☐ ☐ ☐ ☐ ☐ ☐ ☐ ☐

Meal 4   Time:

Food / Beverage	Cals	Carbs	Fat	Protein
Subtotals				

Meal 5   Time:

Food / Beverage	Cals	Carbs	Fat	Protein
Subtotals				

Cals	Carbs	Fat	Protein	Weight

Notes / Excercise

Date _____   Su   Mo   Tu   We   Th   Fr   Sa

Meal 1   Time:

Food / Beverage	Cals	Carbs	Fat	Protein
Subtotals				

Meal 2   Time:

Food / Beverage	Cals	Carbs	Fat	Protein
Subtotals				

Meal 3   Time:

Food / Beverage	Cals	Carbs	Fat	Protein
Subtotals				

8 oz. servings of water ☐ ☐ ☐ ☐ ☐ ☐ ☐ ☐

Meal 4   Time:

Food / Beverage	Cals	Carbs	Fat	Protein
Subtotals				

Meal 5   Time:

Food / Beverage	Cals	Carbs	Fat	Protein
Subtotals				

Cals	Carbs	Fat	Protein	Weight

Notes / Excercise

_____

_____

_____

Date _____   Su   Mo   Tu   We   Th   Fr   Sa

Meal 1   **Time:**

Food / Beverage	Cals	Carbs	Fat	Protein
Subtotals				

Meal 2   **Time:**

Food / Beverage	Cals	Carbs	Fat	Protein
Subtotals				

Meal 3   **Time:**

Food / Beverage	Cals	Carbs	Fat	Protein
Subtotals				

8 oz. servings of water ☐ ☐ ☐ ☐ ☐ ☐ ☐ ☐

Meal 4   Time:

Food / Beverage	Cals	Carbs	Fat	Protein
Subtotals				

Meal 5   Time:

Food / Beverage	Cals	Carbs	Fat	Protein
Subtotals				

Cals	Carbs	Fat	Protein

Weight

Notes / Excercise

_____

_____

_____

Date _____   Su   Mo   Tu   We   Th   Fr   Sa

Meal 1   **Time:**

Food / Beverage	Cals	Carbs	Fat	Protein
Subtotals				

Meal 2   **Time:**

Food / Beverage	Cals	Carbs	Fat	Protein
Subtotals				

Meal 3   **Time:**

Food / Beverage	Cals	Carbs	Fat	Protein
Subtotals				

8 oz. servings of water ☐ ☐ ☐ ☐ ☐ ☐ ☐ ☐

Meal 4   Time:

Food / Beverage	Cals	Carbs	Fat	Protein
Subtotals				

Meal 5   Time:

Food / Beverage	Cals	Carbs	Fat	Protein
Subtotals				

Cals	Carbs	Fat	Protein	Weight

Notes / Excercise

Date _____   Su   Mo   Tu   We   Th   Fr   Sa

Meal 1   **Time:**

Food / Beverage	Cals	Carbs	Fat	Protein
Subtotals				

Meal 2   **Time:**

Food / Beverage	Cals	Carbs	Fat	Protein
Subtotals				

Meal 3   **Time:**

Food / Beverage	Cals	Carbs	Fat	Protein
Subtotals				

8 oz. servings of water ☐ ☐ ☐ ☐ ☐ ☐ ☐ ☐

Meal 4   Time:

Food / Beverage	Cals	Carbs	Fat	Protein
Subtotals				

Meal 5   Time:

Food / Beverage	Cals	Carbs	Fat	Protein
Subtotals				

Cals	Carbs	Fat	Protein		Weight

Notes / Excercise

Date _____   Su   Mo   Tu   We   Th   Fr   Sa

Meal 1   **Time:**

Food / Beverage	Cals	Carbs	Fat	Protein
Subtotals				

Meal 2   **Time:**

Food / Beverage	Cals	Carbs	Fat	Protein
Subtotals				

Meal 3   **Time:**

Food / Beverage	Cals	Carbs	Fat	Protein
Subtotals				

8 oz. servings of water ☐ ☐ ☐ ☐ ☐ ☐ ☐ ☐

Meal 4   Time:

Food / Beverage	Cals	Carbs	Fat	Protein
Subtotals				

Meal 5   Time:

Food / Beverage	Cals	Carbs	Fat	Protein
Subtotals				

Cals	Carbs	Fat	Protein		Weight

Notes / Excercise

_____

_____

_____

Date _____   Su   Mo   Tu   We   Th   Fr   Sa

Meal 1   **Time:**

Food / Beverage	Cals	Carbs	Fat	Protein
Subtotals				

Meal 2   **Time:**

Food / Beverage	Cals	Carbs	Fat	Protein
Subtotals				

Meal 3   **Time:**

Food / Beverage	Cals	Carbs	Fat	Protein
Subtotals				

8 oz. servings of water ☐ ☐ ☐ ☐ ☐ ☐ ☐ ☐

Meal 4   Time:

Food / Beverage	Cals	Carbs	Fat	Protein
Subtotals				

Meal 5   Time:

Food / Beverage	Cals	Carbs	Fat	Protein
Subtotals				

Cals	Carbs	Fat	Protein		Weight

Notes / Excercise

Date _____   Su   Mo   Tu   We   Th   Fr   Sa

Meal 1   **Time:**

Food / Beverage	Cals	Carbs	Fat	Protein
Subtotals				

Meal 2   **Time:**

Food / Beverage	Cals	Carbs	Fat	Protein
Subtotals				

Meal 3   **Time:**

Food / Beverage	Cals	Carbs	Fat	Protein
Subtotals				

8 oz. servings of water ☐ ☐ ☐ ☐ ☐ ☐ ☐ ☐

Meal 4   Time:

Food / Beverage	Cals	Carbs	Fat	Protein
Subtotals				

Meal 5   Time:

Food / Beverage	Cals	Carbs	Fat	Protein
Subtotals				

Cals	Carbs	Fat	Protein		Weight

Notes / Excercise

Date _____   Su   Mo   Tu   We   Th   Fr   Sa

Meal 1   **Time:**

Food / Beverage	Cals	Carbs	Fat	Protein
Subtotals				

Meal 2   **Time:**

Food / Beverage	Cals	Carbs	Fat	Protein
Subtotals				

Meal 3   **Time:**

Food / Beverage	Cals	Carbs	Fat	Protein
Subtotals				

8 oz. servings of water ☐ ☐ ☐ ☐ ☐ ☐ ☐ ☐

Meal 4   Time:

Food / Beverage	Cals	Carbs	Fat	Protein
Subtotals				

Meal 5   Time:

Food / Beverage	Cals	Carbs	Fat	Protein
Subtotals				

Cals	Carbs	Fat	Protein

Weight

Notes / Excercise

_____

_____

_____

Date _____   Su   Mo   Tu   We   Th   Fr   Sa

Meal 1   **Time:**

Food / Beverage	Cals	Carbs	Fat	Protein
Subtotals				

Meal 2   **Time:**

Food / Beverage	Cals	Carbs	Fat	Protein
Subtotals				

Meal 3   **Time:**

Food / Beverage	Cals	Carbs	Fat	Protein
Subtotals				

8 oz. servings of water ☐ ☐ ☐ ☐ ☐ ☐ ☐ ☐

Meal 4   Time:

Food / Beverage	Cals	Carbs	Fat	Protein
Subtotals				

Meal 5   Time:

Food / Beverage	Cals	Carbs	Fat	Protein
Subtotals				

Cals	Carbs	Fat	Protein		Weight

Notes / Excercise

_____

_____

_____

Date _____   Su   Mo   Tu   We   Th   Fr   Sa

Meal 1   **Time:**

Food / Beverage	Cals	Carbs	Fat	Protein
Subtotals				

Meal 2   **Time:**

Food / Beverage	Cals	Carbs	Fat	Protein
Subtotals				

Meal 3   **Time:**

Food / Beverage	Cals	Carbs	Fat	Protein
Subtotals				

8 oz. servings of water ☐ ☐ ☐ ☐ ☐ ☐ ☐ ☐

Meal 4   Time:

Food / Beverage	Cals	Carbs	Fat	Protein
Subtotals				

Meal 5   Time:

Food / Beverage	Cals	Carbs	Fat	Protein
Subtotals				

Cals	Carbs	Fat	Protein		Weight

Notes / Excercise
_____
_____
_____

Date _____   Su   Mo   Tu   We   Th   Fr   Sa

Meal 1   **Time:**

Food / Beverage	Cals	Carbs	Fat	Protein
Subtotals				

Meal 2   **Time:**

Food / Beverage	Cals	Carbs	Fat	Protein
Subtotals				

Meal 3   **Time:**

Food / Beverage	Cals	Carbs	Fat	Protein
Subtotals				

8 oz. servings of water ☐ ☐ ☐ ☐ ☐ ☐ ☐ ☐

Meal 4   Time:

Food / Beverage	Cals	Carbs	Fat	Protein
Subtotals				

Meal 5   Time:

Food / Beverage	Cals	Carbs	Fat	Protein
Subtotals				

Cals	Carbs	Fat	Protein	Weight

Notes / Excercise

Date _____   Su   Mo   Tu   We   Th   Fr   Sa

Meal 1   **Time:**

Food / Beverage	Cals	Carbs	Fat	Protein
Subtotals				

Meal 2   **Time:**

Food / Beverage	Cals	Carbs	Fat	Protein
Subtotals				

Meal 3   **Time:**

Food / Beverage	Cals	Carbs	Fat	Protein
Subtotals				

8 oz. servings of water ☐ ☐ ☐ ☐ ☐ ☐ ☐ ☐

Meal 4   Time:

Food / Beverage	Cals	Carbs	Fat	Protein
Subtotals				

Meal 5   Time:

Food / Beverage	Cals	Carbs	Fat	Protein
Subtotals				

Cals	Carbs	Fat	Protein		Weight

Notes / Excercise

_____

_____

_____

Date _____   Su   Mo   Tu   We   Th   Fr   Sa

Meal 1   **Time:**

Food / Beverage	Cals	Carbs	Fat	Protein
Subtotals				

Meal 2   **Time:**

Food / Beverage	Cals	Carbs	Fat	Protein
Subtotals				

Meal 3   **Time:**

Food / Beverage	Cals	Carbs	Fat	Protein
Subtotals				

8 oz. servings of water ☐ ☐ ☐ ☐ ☐ ☐ ☐ ☐

Meal 4   **Time:**

Food / Beverage	Cals	Carbs	Fat	Protein
Subtotals				

Meal 5   **Time:**

Food / Beverage	Cals	Carbs	Fat	Protein
Subtotals				

Cals	Carbs	Fat	Protein

Weight

Notes / Excercise

_____

_____

_____

Date _____   Su   Mo   Tu   We   Th   Fr   Sa

Meal 1   Time:

Food / Beverage	Cals	Carbs	Fat	Protein
Subtotals				

Meal 2   Time:

Food / Beverage	Cals	Carbs	Fat	Protein
Subtotals				

Meal 3   Time:

Food / Beverage	Cals	Carbs	Fat	Protein
Subtotals				

8 oz. servings of water ☐ ☐ ☐ ☐ ☐ ☐ ☐ ☐

Meal 4   Time:

Food / Beverage	Cals	Carbs	Fat	Protein
Subtotals				

Meal 5   Time:

Food / Beverage	Cals	Carbs	Fat	Protein
Subtotals				

Cals	Carbs	Fat	Protein		Weight

Notes / Excercise

Date _____   Su   Mo   Tu   We   Th   Fr   Sa

Meal 1   Time:

Food / Beverage	Cals	Carbs	Fat	Protein
Subtotals				

Meal 2   Time:

Food / Beverage	Cals	Carbs	Fat	Protein
Subtotals				

Meal 3   Time:

Food / Beverage	Cals	Carbs	Fat	Protein
Subtotals				

8 oz. servings of water ☐ ☐ ☐ ☐ ☐ ☐ ☐ ☐

Meal 4   Time:

Food / Beverage	Cals	Carbs	Fat	Protein
Subtotals				

Meal 5   Time:

Food / Beverage	Cals	Carbs	Fat	Protein
Subtotals				

Cals	Carbs	Fat	Protein

Weight

Notes / Excercise

Date _____   Su   Mo   Tu   We   Th   Fr   Sa

Meal 1   **Time:**

Food / Beverage	Cals	Carbs	Fat	Protein
Subtotals				

Meal 2   **Time:**

Food / Beverage	Cals	Carbs	Fat	Protein
Subtotals				

Meal 3   **Time:**

Food / Beverage	Cals	Carbs	Fat	Protein
Subtotals				

8 oz. servings of water ☐ ☐ ☐ ☐ ☐ ☐ ☐ ☐

Meal 4   Time:

Food / Beverage	Cals	Carbs	Fat	Protein
Subtotals				

Meal 5   Time:

Food / Beverage	Cals	Carbs	Fat	Protein
Subtotals				

Cals	Carbs	Fat	Protein		Weight

Notes / Excercise

_____

_____

_____

Date _____   Su   Mo   Tu   We   Th   Fr   Sa

Meal 1   **Time:**

Food / Beverage	Cals	Carbs	Fat	Protein
Subtotals				

Meal 2   **Time:**

Food / Beverage	Cals	Carbs	Fat	Protein
Subtotals				

Meal 3   **Time:**

Food / Beverage	Cals	Carbs	Fat	Protein
Subtotals				

8 oz. servings of water ☐ ☐ ☐ ☐ ☐ ☐ ☐ ☐

Meal 4   Time:

Food / Beverage	Cals	Carbs	Fat	Protein
Subtotals				

Meal 5   Time:

Food / Beverage	Cals	Carbs	Fat	Protein
Subtotals				

Cals	Carbs	Fat	Protein

Weight

Notes / Excercise

Date _____   Su   Mo   Tu   We   Th   Fr   Sa

Meal 1   **Time:**

Food / Beverage	Cals	Carbs	Fat	Protein
Subtotals				

Meal 2   **Time:**

Food / Beverage	Cals	Carbs	Fat	Protein
Subtotals				

Meal 3   **Time:**

Food / Beverage	Cals	Carbs	Fat	Protein
Subtotals				

8 oz. servings of water ☐ ☐ ☐ ☐ ☐ ☐ ☐ ☐

Meal 4   Time:

Food / Beverage	Cals	Carbs	Fat	Protein
Subtotals				

Meal 5   Time:

Food / Beverage	Cals	Carbs	Fat	Protein
Subtotals				

Cals	Carbs	Fat	Protein

Weight

Notes / Excercise

Date _____   Su   Mo   Tu   We   Th   Fr   Sa

Meal 1   Time:

Food / Beverage	Cals	Carbs	Fat	Protein
Subtotals				

Meal 2   Time:

Food / Beverage	Cals	Carbs	Fat	Protein
Subtotals				

Meal 3   Time:

Food / Beverage	Cals	Carbs	Fat	Protein
Subtotals				

8 oz. servings of water ☐ ☐ ☐ ☐ ☐ ☐ ☐ ☐

Meal 4   Time:

Food / Beverage	Cals	Carbs	Fat	Protein
Subtotals				

Meal 5   Time:

Food / Beverage	Cals	Carbs	Fat	Protein
Subtotals				

Cals	Carbs	Fat	Protein		Weight

Notes / Excercise

Date _____   Su   Mo   Tu   We   Th   Fr   Sa

Meal 1   **Time:**

Food / Beverage	Cals	Carbs	Fat	Protein
Subtotals				

Meal 2   **Time:**

Food / Beverage	Cals	Carbs	Fat	Protein
Subtotals				

Meal 3   **Time:**

Food / Beverage	Cals	Carbs	Fat	Protein
Subtotals				

8 oz. servings of water ☐ ☐ ☐ ☐ ☐ ☐ ☐ ☐

Meal 4   Time:

Food / Beverage	Cals	Carbs	Fat	Protein
Subtotals				

Meal 5   Time:

Food / Beverage	Cals	Carbs	Fat	Protein
Subtotals				

Cals	Carbs	Fat	Protein

Weight

Notes / Excercise

_____

_____

_____

Date _____   Su   Mo   Tu   We   Th   Fr   Sa

Meal 1   **Time:**

Food / Beverage	Cals	Carbs	Fat	Protein
Subtotals				

Meal 2   **Time:**

Food / Beverage	Cals	Carbs	Fat	Protein
Subtotals				

Meal 3   **Time:**

Food / Beverage	Cals	Carbs	Fat	Protein
Subtotals				

8 oz. servings of water ☐ ☐ ☐ ☐ ☐ ☐ ☐ ☐

Meal 4   Time:

Food / Beverage	Cals	Carbs	Fat	Protein
Subtotals				

Meal 5   Time:

Food / Beverage	Cals	Carbs	Fat	Protein
Subtotals				

Cals	Carbs	Fat	Protein	Weight

Notes / Excercise

_____

_____

_____

Date _____   Su   Mo   Tu   We   Th   Fr   Sa

Meal 1   **Time:**

Food / Beverage	Cals	Carbs	Fat	Protein
Subtotals				

Meal 2   **Time:**

Food / Beverage	Cals	Carbs	Fat	Protein
Subtotals				

Meal 3   **Time:**

Food / Beverage	Cals	Carbs	Fat	Protein
Subtotals				

8 oz. servings of water ☐ ☐ ☐ ☐ ☐ ☐ ☐ ☐

Meal 4   **Time:**

Food / Beverage	Cals	Carbs	Fat	Protein
Subtotals				

Meal 5   **Time:**

Food / Beverage	Cals	Carbs	Fat	Protein
Subtotals				

Cals	Carbs	Fat	Protein

Weight

Notes / Excercise

Date _____   Su   Mo   Tu   We   Th   Fr   Sa

Meal 1   **Time:**

Food / Beverage	Cals	Carbs	Fat	Protein
Subtotals				

Meal 2   **Time:**

Food / Beverage	Cals	Carbs	Fat	Protein
Subtotals				

Meal 3   **Time:**

Food / Beverage	Cals	Carbs	Fat	Protein
Subtotals				

8 oz. servings of water ☐ ☐ ☐ ☐ ☐ ☐ ☐ ☐

Meal 4   Time:

Food / Beverage	Cals	Carbs	Fat	Protein
Subtotals				

Meal 5   Time:

Food / Beverage	Cals	Carbs	Fat	Protein
Subtotals				

Cals	Carbs	Fat	Protein		Weight

Notes / Excercise

Date _____   Su   Mo   Tu   We   Th   Fr   Sa

Meal 1   **Time:**

Food / Beverage	Cals	Carbs	Fat	Protein
Subtotals				

Meal 2   **Time:**

Food / Beverage	Cals	Carbs	Fat	Protein
Subtotals				

Meal 3   **Time:**

Food / Beverage	Cals	Carbs	Fat	Protein
Subtotals				

8 oz. servings of water ☐ ☐ ☐ ☐ ☐ ☐ ☐ ☐

Meal 4   Time:

Food / Beverage	Cals	Carbs	Fat	Protein
Subtotals				

Meal 5   Time:

Food / Beverage	Cals	Carbs	Fat	Protein
Subtotals				

Cals	Carbs	Fat	Protein		Weight

Notes / Excercise

_____

_____

_____

Date _____   Su   Mo   Tu   We   Th   Fr   Sa

Meal 1   Time:

Food / Beverage	Cals	Carbs	Fat	Protein
Subtotals				

Meal 2   Time:

Food / Beverage	Cals	Carbs	Fat	Protein
Subtotals				

Meal 3   Time:

Food / Beverage	Cals	Carbs	Fat	Protein
Subtotals				

8 oz. servings of water ☐ ☐ ☐ ☐ ☐ ☐ ☐ ☐

Meal 4   Time:

Food / Beverage	Cals	Carbs	Fat	Protein
Subtotals				

Meal 5   Time:

Food / Beverage	Cals	Carbs	Fat	Protein
Subtotals				

Cals	Carbs	Fat	Protein	Weight

Notes / Excercise
_____
_____
_____

Date _____   Su   Mo   Tu   We   Th   Fr   Sa

Meal 1   **Time:**

Food / Beverage	Cals	Carbs	Fat	Protein
Subtotals				

Meal 2   **Time:**

Food / Beverage	Cals	Carbs	Fat	Protein
Subtotals				

Meal 3   **Time:**

Food / Beverage	Cals	Carbs	Fat	Protein
Subtotals				

8 oz. servings of water ☐ ☐ ☐ ☐ ☐ ☐ ☐ ☐

Meal 4   Time:

Food / Beverage	Cals	Carbs	Fat	Protein
Subtotals				

Meal 5   Time:

Food / Beverage	Cals	Carbs	Fat	Protein
Subtotals				

Cals	Carbs	Fat	Protein

Weight

Notes / Excercise

Date _____   Su   Mo   Tu   We   Th   Fr   Sa

Meal 1   **Time:**

Food / Beverage	Cals	Carbs	Fat	Protein
Subtotals				

Meal 2   **Time:**

Food / Beverage	Cals	Carbs	Fat	Protein
Subtotals				

Meal 3   **Time:**

Food / Beverage	Cals	Carbs	Fat	Protein
Subtotals				

8 oz. servings of water ☐ ☐ ☐ ☐ ☐ ☐ ☐ ☐

Meal 4   **Time:**

Food / Beverage	Cals	Carbs	Fat	Protein
Subtotals				

Meal 5   **Time:**

Food / Beverage	Cals	Carbs	Fat	Protein
Subtotals				

Cals	Carbs	Fat	Protein

Weight

Notes / Excercise

_____

_____

_____

Date _____   Su   Mo   Tu   We   Th   Fr   Sa

Meal 1   **Time:**

Food / Beverage	Cals	Carbs	Fat	Protein
Subtotals				

Meal 2   **Time:**

Food / Beverage	Cals	Carbs	Fat	Protein
Subtotals				

Meal 3   **Time:**

Food / Beverage	Cals	Carbs	Fat	Protein
Subtotals				

8 oz. servings of water ☐ ☐ ☐ ☐ ☐ ☐ ☐ ☐

Meal 4   Time:

Food / Beverage	Cals	Carbs	Fat	Protein
Subtotals				

Meal 5   Time:

Food / Beverage	Cals	Carbs	Fat	Protein
Subtotals				

Cals	Carbs	Fat	Protein		Weight

Notes / Excercise

Date _____   Su   Mo   Tu   We   Th   Fr   Sa

Meal 1   Time:

Food / Beverage	Cals	Carbs	Fat	Protein
Subtotals				

Meal 2   Time:

Food / Beverage	Cals	Carbs	Fat	Protein
Subtotals				

Meal 3   Time:

Food / Beverage	Cals	Carbs	Fat	Protein
Subtotals				

8 oz. servings of water ☐ ☐ ☐ ☐ ☐ ☐ ☐ ☐

Meal 4   Time:

Food / Beverage	Cals	Carbs	Fat	Protein
Subtotals				

Meal 5   Time:

Food / Beverage	Cals	Carbs	Fat	Protein
Subtotals				

Cals	Carbs	Fat	Protein	Weight

Notes / Excercise

Date _____   Su   Mo   Tu   We   Th   Fr   Sa

Meal 1   **Time:**

Food / Beverage	Cals	Carbs	Fat	Protein
Subtotals				

Meal 2   **Time:**

Food / Beverage	Cals	Carbs	Fat	Protein
Subtotals				

Meal 3   **Time:**

Food / Beverage	Cals	Carbs	Fat	Protein
Subtotals				

8 oz. servings of water ☐ ☐ ☐ ☐ ☐ ☐ ☐ ☐

Meal 4   Time:

Food / Beverage	Cals	Carbs	Fat	Protein
Subtotals				

Meal 5   Time:

Food / Beverage	Cals	Carbs	Fat	Protein
Subtotals				

Cals	Carbs	Fat	Protein	Weight

Notes / Excercise

Date _____   Su   Mo   Tu   We   Th   Fr   Sa

Meal 1   **Time:**

Food / Beverage	Cals	Carbs	Fat	Protein
Subtotals				

Meal 2   **Time:**

Food / Beverage	Cals	Carbs	Fat	Protein
Subtotals				

Meal 3   **Time:**

Food / Beverage	Cals	Carbs	Fat	Protein
Subtotals				

8 oz. servings of water ☐ ☐ ☐ ☐ ☐ ☐ ☐ ☐

Meal 4   Time:

Food / Beverage	Cals	Carbs	Fat	Protein
Subtotals				

Meal 5   Time:

Food / Beverage	Cals	Carbs	Fat	Protein
Subtotals				

Cals	Carbs	Fat	Protein

Weight

Notes / Excercise

_____

_____

_____

Date _____   Su   Mo   Tu   We   Th   Fr   Sa

Meal 1   **Time:**

Food / Beverage	Cals	Carbs	Fat	Protein
Subtotals				

Meal 2   **Time:**

Food / Beverage	Cals	Carbs	Fat	Protein
Subtotals				

Meal 3   **Time:**

Food / Beverage	Cals	Carbs	Fat	Protein
Subtotals				

8 oz. servings of water ☐ ☐ ☐ ☐ ☐ ☐ ☐ ☐

Meal 4   Time:

Food / Beverage	Cals	Carbs	Fat	Protein
Subtotals				

Meal 5   Time:

Food / Beverage	Cals	Carbs	Fat	Protein
Subtotals				

Cals	Carbs	Fat	Protein		Weight

Notes / Excercise

Date _____   Su   Mo   Tu   We   Th   Fr   Sa

Meal 1   **Time:**

Food / Beverage	Cals	Carbs	Fat	Protein
Subtotals				

Meal 2   **Time:**

Food / Beverage	Cals	Carbs	Fat	Protein
Subtotals				

Meal 3   **Time:**

Food / Beverage	Cals	Carbs	Fat	Protein
Subtotals				

8 oz. servings of water ☐ ☐ ☐ ☐ ☐ ☐ ☐ ☐

Meal 4   Time:

Food / Beverage	Cals	Carbs	Fat	Protein
Subtotals				

Meal 5   Time:

Food / Beverage	Cals	Carbs	Fat	Protein
Subtotals				

Cals	Carbs	Fat	Protein		Weight

Notes / Excercise

_____

_____

_____

Date _____   Su   Mo   Tu   We   Th   Fr   Sa

Meal 1   Time:

Food / Beverage	Cals	Carbs	Fat	Protein
Subtotals				

Meal 2   Time:

Food / Beverage	Cals	Carbs	Fat	Protein
Subtotals				

Meal 3   Time:

Food / Beverage	Cals	Carbs	Fat	Protein
Subtotals				

8 oz. servings of water ☐ ☐ ☐ ☐ ☐ ☐ ☐ ☐

Meal 4   Time:

Food / Beverage	Cals	Carbs	Fat	Protein
Subtotals				

Meal 5   Time:

Food / Beverage	Cals	Carbs	Fat	Protein
Subtotals				

Cals	Carbs	Fat	Protein		Weight

Notes / Excercise

Date _____   Su   Mo   Tu   We   Th   Fr   Sa

Meal 1   **Time:**

Food / Beverage	Cals	Carbs	Fat	Protein
Subtotals				

Meal 2   **Time:**

Food / Beverage	Cals	Carbs	Fat	Protein
Subtotals				

Meal 3   **Time:**

Food / Beverage	Cals	Carbs	Fat	Protein
Subtotals				

8 oz. servings of water ☐ ☐ ☐ ☐ ☐ ☐ ☐ ☐

Meal 4   Time:

Food / Beverage	Cals	Carbs	Fat	Protein
Subtotals				

Meal 5   Time:

Food / Beverage	Cals	Carbs	Fat	Protein
Subtotals				

Cals	Carbs	Fat	Protein

Weight

Notes / Excercise

_____

_____

Date _____   Su   Mo   Tu   We   Th   Fr   Sa

Meal 1   **Time:**

Food / Beverage	Cals	Carbs	Fat	Protein
Subtotals				

Meal 2   **Time:**

Food / Beverage	Cals	Carbs	Fat	Protein
Subtotals				

Meal 3   **Time:**

Food / Beverage	Cals	Carbs	Fat	Protein
Subtotals				

8 oz. servings of water ☐ ☐ ☐ ☐ ☐ ☐ ☐ ☐

Meal 4   Time:

Food / Beverage	Cals	Carbs	Fat	Protein
Subtotals				

Meal 5   Time:

Food / Beverage	Cals	Carbs	Fat	Protein
Subtotals				

Cals	Carbs	Fat	Protein

Weight

Notes / Excercise

Date _____ Su Mo Tu We Th Fr Sa

Meal 1   Time:

Food / Beverage	Cals	Carbs	Fat	Protein
Subtotals				

Meal 2   Time:

Food / Beverage	Cals	Carbs	Fat	Protein
Subtotals				

Meal 3   Time:

Food / Beverage	Cals	Carbs	Fat	Protein
Subtotals				

8 oz. servings of water ☐ ☐ ☐ ☐ ☐ ☐ ☐ ☐

Meal 4   Time:

Food / Beverage	Cals	Carbs	Fat	Protein
Subtotals				

Meal 5   Time:

Food / Beverage	Cals	Carbs	Fat	Protein
Subtotals				

Cals	Carbs	Fat	Protein

Weight

Notes / Excercise

_____

_____

_____

Date _____   Su   Mo   Tu   We   Th   Fr   Sa

Meal 1   **Time:**

Food / Beverage	Cals	Carbs	Fat	Protein
Subtotals				

Meal 2   **Time:**

Food / Beverage	Cals	Carbs	Fat	Protein
Subtotals				

Meal 3   **Time:**

Food / Beverage	Cals	Carbs	Fat	Protein
Subtotals				

8 oz. servings of water ☐ ☐ ☐ ☐ ☐ ☐ ☐ ☐

Meal 4   Time:

Food / Beverage	Cals	Carbs	Fat	Protein
Subtotals				

Meal 5   Time:

Food / Beverage	Cals	Carbs	Fat	Protein
Subtotals				

Cals	Carbs	Fat	Protein		Weight

Notes / Excercise

Date _____   Su   Mo   Tu   We   Th   Fr   Sa

Meal 1   **Time:**

Food / Beverage	Cals	Carbs	Fat	Protein
Subtotals				

Meal 2   **Time:**

Food / Beverage	Cals	Carbs	Fat	Protein
Subtotals				

Meal 3   **Time:**

Food / Beverage	Cals	Carbs	Fat	Protein
Subtotals				

8 oz. servings of water ☐ ☐ ☐ ☐ ☐ ☐ ☐ ☐

Meal 4   Time:

Food / Beverage	Cals	Carbs	Fat	Protein
Subtotals				

Meal 5   Time:

Food / Beverage	Cals	Carbs	Fat	Protein
Subtotals				

Cals	Carbs	Fat	Protein

Weight

Notes / Excercise

Date _____   Su   Mo   Tu   We   Th   Fr   Sa

Meal 1   **Time:**

Food / Beverage	Cals	Carbs	Fat	Protein
Subtotals				

Meal 2   **Time:**

Food / Beverage	Cals	Carbs	Fat	Protein
Subtotals				

Meal 3   **Time:**

Food / Beverage	Cals	Carbs	Fat	Protein
Subtotals				

8 oz. servings of water ☐ ☐ ☐ ☐ ☐ ☐ ☐ ☐

Meal 4   Time:

Food / Beverage	Cals	Carbs	Fat	Protein
Subtotals				

Meal 5   Time:

Food / Beverage	Cals	Carbs	Fat	Protein
Subtotals				

Cals	Carbs	Fat	Protein	Weight

Notes / Excercise

_____

_____

_____

Date _____   Su   Mo   Tu   We   Th   Fr   Sa

Meal 1   **Time:**

Food / Beverage	Cals	Carbs	Fat	Protein
Subtotals				

Meal 2   **Time:**

Food / Beverage	Cals	Carbs	Fat	Protein
Subtotals				

Meal 3   **Time:**

Food / Beverage	Cals	Carbs	Fat	Protein
Subtotals				

8 oz. servings of water ☐ ☐ ☐ ☐ ☐ ☐ ☐ ☐

Meal 4   Time:

Food / Beverage	Cals	Carbs	Fat	Protein
Subtotals				

Meal 5   Time:

Food / Beverage	Cals	Carbs	Fat	Protein
Subtotals				

Cals	Carbs	Fat	Protein	Weight

Notes / Excercise

Date _____   Su   Mo   Tu   We   Th   Fr   Sa

Meal 1   **Time:**

Food / Beverage	Cals	Carbs	Fat	Protein
Subtotals				

Meal 2   **Time:**

Food / Beverage	Cals	Carbs	Fat	Protein
Subtotals				

Meal 3   **Time:**

Food / Beverage	Cals	Carbs	Fat	Protein
Subtotals				

8 oz. servings of water ☐ ☐ ☐ ☐ ☐ ☐ ☐ ☐

Meal 4   Time:

Food / Beverage	Cals	Carbs	Fat	Protein
Subtotals				

Meal 5   Time:

Food / Beverage	Cals	Carbs	Fat	Protein
Subtotals				

Cals	Carbs	Fat	Protein	Weight

Notes / Excercise

_____

_____

_____

Date _____   Su   Mo   Tu   We   Th   Fr   Sa

Meal 1   Time:

Food / Beverage	Cals	Carbs	Fat	Protein
Subtotals				

Meal 2   Time:

Food / Beverage	Cals	Carbs	Fat	Protein
Subtotals				

Meal 3   Time:

Food / Beverage	Cals	Carbs	Fat	Protein
Subtotals				

8 oz. servings of water ☐ ☐ ☐ ☐ ☐ ☐ ☐ ☐

Meal 4   Time:

Food / Beverage	Cals	Carbs	Fat	Protein
Subtotals				

Meal 5   Time:

Food / Beverage	Cals	Carbs	Fat	Protein
Subtotals				

Cals	Carbs	Fat	Protein		Weight

Notes / Excercise
_____
_____
_____

Date _____   Su   Mo   Tu   We   Th   Fr   Sa

Meal 1   **Time:**

Food / Beverage	Cals	Carbs	Fat	Protein
Subtotals				

Meal 2   **Time:**

Food / Beverage	Cals	Carbs	Fat	Protein
Subtotals				

Meal 3   **Time:**

Food / Beverage	Cals	Carbs	Fat	Protein
Subtotals				

8 oz. servings of water ☐ ☐ ☐ ☐ ☐ ☐ ☐ ☐

Meal 4   Time:

Food / Beverage	Cals	Carbs	Fat	Protein
Subtotals				

Meal 5   Time:

Food / Beverage	Cals	Carbs	Fat	Protein
Subtotals				

Cals	Carbs	Fat	Protein

Weight

Notes / Excercise

Date _____   Su   Mo   Tu   We   Th   Fr   Sa

Meal 1   Time:

Food / Beverage	Cals	Carbs	Fat	Protein
Subtotals				

Meal 2   Time:

Food / Beverage	Cals	Carbs	Fat	Protein
Subtotals				

Meal 3   Time:

Food / Beverage	Cals	Carbs	Fat	Protein
Subtotals				

8 oz. servings of water ☐ ☐ ☐ ☐ ☐ ☐ ☐ ☐

Meal 4   Time:

Food / Beverage	Cals	Carbs	Fat	Protein
Subtotals				

Meal 5   Time:

Food / Beverage	Cals	Carbs	Fat	Protein
Subtotals				

Cals	Carbs	Fat	Protein	Weight

Notes / Excercise

_____

_____

_____

Date _____   Su   Mo   Tu   We   Th   Fr   Sa

Meal 1   **Time:**

Food / Beverage	Cals	Carbs	Fat	Protein
Subtotals				

Meal 2   **Time:**

Food / Beverage	Cals	Carbs	Fat	Protein
Subtotals				

Meal 3   **Time:**

Food / Beverage	Cals	Carbs	Fat	Protein
Subtotals				

8 oz. servings of water ☐ ☐ ☐ ☐ ☐ ☐ ☐ ☐

Meal 4   Time:

Food / Beverage	Cals	Carbs	Fat	Protein
Subtotals				

Meal 5   Time:

Food / Beverage	Cals	Carbs	Fat	Protein
Subtotals				

Cals	Carbs	Fat	Protein	Weight

Notes / Excercise

Date _____   Su   Mo   Tu   We   Th   Fr   Sa

Meal 1   Time:

Food / Beverage	Cals	Carbs	Fat	Protein
Subtotals				

Meal 2   Time:

Food / Beverage	Cals	Carbs	Fat	Protein
Subtotals				

Meal 3   Time:

Food / Beverage	Cals	Carbs	Fat	Protein
Subtotals				

8 oz. servings of water ☐ ☐ ☐ ☐ ☐ ☐ ☐ ☐

Meal 4   Time:

Food / Beverage	Cals	Carbs	Fat	Protein
Subtotals				

Meal 5   Time:

Food / Beverage	Cals	Carbs	Fat	Protein
Subtotals				

Cals	Carbs	Fat	Protein	Weight

Notes / Excercise
_____
_____
_____

Date _____   Su   Mo   Tu   We   Th   Fr   Sa

Meal 1   **Time:**

Food / Beverage	Cals	Carbs	Fat	Protein
Subtotals				

Meal 2   **Time:**

Food / Beverage	Cals	Carbs	Fat	Protein
Subtotals				

Meal 3   **Time:**

Food / Beverage	Cals	Carbs	Fat	Protein
Subtotals				

8 oz. servings of water ☐ ☐ ☐ ☐ ☐ ☐ ☐ ☐

Meal 4   Time:

Food / Beverage	Cals	Carbs	Fat	Protein
Subtotals				

Meal 5   Time:

Food / Beverage	Cals	Carbs	Fat	Protein
Subtotals				

Cals	Carbs	Fat	Protein	Weight

Notes / Excercise
_____

_____

_____

Date _____   Su   Mo   Tu   We   Th   Fr   Sa

Meal 1   Time:

Food / Beverage	Cals	Carbs	Fat	Protein
Subtotals				

Meal 2   Time:

Food / Beverage	Cals	Carbs	Fat	Protein
Subtotals				

Meal 3   Time:

Food / Beverage	Cals	Carbs	Fat	Protein
Subtotals				

8 oz. servings of water ☐ ☐ ☐ ☐ ☐ ☐ ☐ ☐

Meal 4   Time:

Food / Beverage	Cals	Carbs	Fat	Protein
Subtotals				

Meal 5   Time:

Food / Beverage	Cals	Carbs	Fat	Protein
Subtotals				

Cals	Carbs	Fat	Protein

Weight

Notes / Excercise

Date _____   Su Mo Tu We Th Fr Sa

Meal 1   **Time:**

Food / Beverage	Cals	Carbs	Fat	Protein
Subtotals				

Meal 2   **Time:**

Food / Beverage	Cals	Carbs	Fat	Protein
Subtotals				

Meal 3   **Time:**

Food / Beverage	Cals	Carbs	Fat	Protein
Subtotals				

8 oz. servings of water ☐ ☐ ☐ ☐ ☐ ☐ ☐ ☐

Meal 4   Time:

Food / Beverage	Cals	Carbs	Fat	Protein
Subtotals				

Meal 5   Time:

Food / Beverage	Cals	Carbs	Fat	Protein
Subtotals				

Cals	Carbs	Fat	Protein

Weight

Notes / Excercise
_____
_____
_____

Date _____   Su   Mo   Tu   We   Th   Fr   Sa

Meal 1   **Time:**

Food / Beverage	Cals	Carbs	Fat	Protein
Subtotals				

Meal 2   **Time:**

Food / Beverage	Cals	Carbs	Fat	Protein
Subtotals				

Meal 3   **Time:**

Food / Beverage	Cals	Carbs	Fat	Protein
Subtotals				

8 oz. servings of water ☐ ☐ ☐ ☐ ☐ ☐ ☐ ☐

Meal 4   Time:

Food / Beverage	Cals	Carbs	Fat	Protein
Subtotals				

Meal 5   Time:

Food / Beverage	Cals	Carbs	Fat	Protein
Subtotals				

Cals	Carbs	Fat	Protein

Weight

Notes / Excercise
_____

_____

_____

Date _____   Su   Mo   Tu   We   Th   Fr   Sa

Meal 1   **Time:**

Food / Beverage	Cals	Carbs	Fat	Protein
Subtotals				

Meal 2   **Time:**

Food / Beverage	Cals	Carbs	Fat	Protein
Subtotals				

Meal 3   **Time:**

Food / Beverage	Cals	Carbs	Fat	Protein
Subtotals				

8 oz. servings of water ☐ ☐ ☐ ☐ ☐ ☐ ☐ ☐

Meal 4   Time:

Food / Beverage	Cals	Carbs	Fat	Protein
Subtotals				

Meal 5   Time:

Food / Beverage	Cals	Carbs	Fat	Protein
Subtotals				

Cals	Carbs	Fat	Protein		Weight

Notes / Excercise

_____

_____

_____

Date _____   Su   Mo   Tu   We   Th   Fr   Sa

Meal 1   Time:

Food / Beverage	Cals	Carbs	Fat	Protein
Subtotals				

Meal 2   Time:

Food / Beverage	Cals	Carbs	Fat	Protein
Subtotals				

Meal 3   Time:

Food / Beverage	Cals	Carbs	Fat	Protein
Subtotals				

8 oz. servings of water ☐ ☐ ☐ ☐ ☐ ☐ ☐ ☐

Meal 4   Time:

Food / Beverage	Cals	Carbs	Fat	Protein
Subtotals				

Meal 5   Time:

Food / Beverage	Cals	Carbs	Fat	Protein
Subtotals				

Cals	Carbs	Fat	Protein	Weight

Notes / Excercise

Date _____   Su   Mo   Tu   We   Th   Fr   Sa

Meal 1   **Time:**

Food / Beverage	Cals	Carbs	Fat	Protein
Subtotals				

Meal 2   **Time:**

Food / Beverage	Cals	Carbs	Fat	Protein
Subtotals				

Meal 3   **Time:**

Food / Beverage	Cals	Carbs	Fat	Protein
Subtotals				

8 oz. servings of water ☐ ☐ ☐ ☐ ☐ ☐ ☐ ☐

Meal 4   Time:

Food / Beverage	Cals	Carbs	Fat	Protein
Subtotals				

Meal 5   Time:

Food / Beverage	Cals	Carbs	Fat	Protein
Subtotals				

Cals	Carbs	Fat	Protein

Weight

Notes / Excercise

Date _____   Su   Mo   Tu   We   Th   Fr   Sa

Meal 1   Time:

Food / Beverage	Cals	Carbs	Fat	Protein
Subtotals				

Meal 2   Time:

Food / Beverage	Cals	Carbs	Fat	Protein
Subtotals				

Meal 3   Time:

Food / Beverage	Cals	Carbs	Fat	Protein
Subtotals				

8 oz. servings of water ☐ ☐ ☐ ☐ ☐ ☐ ☐ ☐

Meal 4   Time:

Food / Beverage	Cals	Carbs	Fat	Protein
Subtotals				

Meal 5   Time:

Food / Beverage	Cals	Carbs	Fat	Protein
Subtotals				

Cals	Carbs	Fat	Protein	Weight

Notes / Excercise

Date _____   Su   Mo   Tu   We   Th   Fr   Sa

Meal 1   **Time:**

Food / Beverage	Cals	Carbs	Fat	Protein
Subtotals				

Meal 2   **Time:**

Food / Beverage	Cals	Carbs	Fat	Protein
Subtotals				

Meal 3   **Time:**

Food / Beverage	Cals	Carbs	Fat	Protein
Subtotals				

8 oz. servings of water ☐ ☐ ☐ ☐ ☐ ☐ ☐ ☐

Meal 4   Time:

Food / Beverage	Cals	Carbs	Fat	Protein
Subtotals				

Meal 5   Time:

Food / Beverage	Cals	Carbs	Fat	Protein
Subtotals				

Cals	Carbs	Fat	Protein	Weight

Notes / Excercise
_____

_____

_____

Date _____   Su   Mo   Tu   We   Th   Fr   Sa

Meal 1   **Time:**

Food / Beverage	Cals	Carbs	Fat	Protein
Subtotals				

Meal 2   **Time:**

Food / Beverage	Cals	Carbs	Fat	Protein
Subtotals				

Meal 3   **Time:**

Food / Beverage	Cals	Carbs	Fat	Protein
Subtotals				

8 oz. servings of water ☐ ☐ ☐ ☐ ☐ ☐ ☐ ☐

Meal 4   Time:

Food / Beverage	Cals	Carbs	Fat	Protein
Subtotals				

Meal 5   Time:

Food / Beverage	Cals	Carbs	Fat	Protein
Subtotals				

Cals	Carbs	Fat	Protein		Weight

Notes / Excercise
_____

_____

_____

Date _____   Su   Mo   Tu   We   Th   Fr   Sa

Meal 1   **Time:**

Food / Beverage	Cals	Carbs	Fat	Protein
Subtotals				

Meal 2   **Time:**

Food / Beverage	Cals	Carbs	Fat	Protein
Subtotals				

Meal 3   **Time:**

Food / Beverage	Cals	Carbs	Fat	Protein
Subtotals				

8 oz. servings of water ☐ ☐ ☐ ☐ ☐ ☐ ☐ ☐

Meal 4   Time:

Food / Beverage	Cals	Carbs	Fat	Protein
Subtotals				

Meal 5   Time:

Food / Beverage	Cals	Carbs	Fat	Protein
Subtotals				

Cals	Carbs	Fat	Protein

Weight

Notes / Excercise

_____

_____

_____

Date _____   Su   Mo   Tu   We   Th   Fr   Sa

Meal 1   Time:

Food / Beverage	Cals	Carbs	Fat	Protein
Subtotals				

Meal 2   Time:

Food / Beverage	Cals	Carbs	Fat	Protein
Subtotals				

Meal 3   Time:

Food / Beverage	Cals	Carbs	Fat	Protein
Subtotals				

8 oz. servings of water ☐ ☐ ☐ ☐ ☐ ☐ ☐ ☐

Meal 4   Time:

Food / Beverage	Cals	Carbs	Fat	Protein
Subtotals				

Meal 5   Time:

Food / Beverage	Cals	Carbs	Fat	Protein
Subtotals				

Cals	Carbs	Fat	Protein	Weight

Notes / Excercise

Date _____   Su   Mo   Tu   We   Th   Fr   Sa

Meal 1   **Time:**

Food / Beverage	Cals	Carbs	Fat	Protein
Subtotals				

Meal 2   **Time:**

Food / Beverage	Cals	Carbs	Fat	Protein
Subtotals				

Meal 3   **Time:**

Food / Beverage	Cals	Carbs	Fat	Protein
Subtotals				

8 oz. servings of water ☐ ☐ ☐ ☐ ☐ ☐ ☐ ☐

Meal 4   Time:

Food / Beverage	Cals	Carbs	Fat	Protein
Subtotals				

Meal 5   Time:

Food / Beverage	Cals	Carbs	Fat	Protein
Subtotals				

Cals	Carbs	Fat	Protein

Weight

Notes / Excercise

_____

_____

_____

Date _____   Su   Mo   Tu   We   Th   Fr   Sa

Meal 1   Time:

Food / Beverage	Cals	Carbs	Fat	Protein
Subtotals				

Meal 2   Time:

Food / Beverage	Cals	Carbs	Fat	Protein
Subtotals				

Meal 3   Time:

Food / Beverage	Cals	Carbs	Fat	Protein
Subtotals				

8 oz. servings of water ☐ ☐ ☐ ☐ ☐ ☐ ☐ ☐

Meal 4   Time:

Food / Beverage	Cals	Carbs	Fat	Protein
Subtotals				

Meal 5   Time:

Food / Beverage	Cals	Carbs	Fat	Protein
Subtotals				

Cals	Carbs	Fat	Protein	Weight

Notes / Excercise

Date _____   Su   Mo   Tu   We   Th   Fr   Sa

Meal 1   **Time:**

Food / Beverage	Cals	Carbs	Fat	Protein
Subtotals				

Meal 2   **Time:**

Food / Beverage	Cals	Carbs	Fat	Protein
Subtotals				

Meal 3   **Time:**

Food / Beverage	Cals	Carbs	Fat	Protein
Subtotals				

8 oz. servings of water ☐ ☐ ☐ ☐ ☐ ☐ ☐ ☐

Meal 4   Time:

Food / Beverage	Cals	Carbs	Fat	Protein
Subtotals				

Meal 5   Time:

Food / Beverage	Cals	Carbs	Fat	Protein
Subtotals				

Cals	Carbs	Fat	Protein

Weight

Notes / Excercise

_____

_____

_____

Date _____   Su   Mo   Tu   We   Th   Fr   Sa

Meal 1   **Time:**

Food / Beverage	Cals	Carbs	Fat	Protein
Subtotals				

Meal 2   **Time:**

Food / Beverage	Cals	Carbs	Fat	Protein
Subtotals				

Meal 3   **Time:**

Food / Beverage	Cals	Carbs	Fat	Protein
Subtotals				

8 oz. servings of water ☐ ☐ ☐ ☐ ☐ ☐ ☐ ☐

Meal 4   Time:

Food / Beverage	Cals	Carbs	Fat	Protein
Subtotals				

Meal 5   Time:

Food / Beverage	Cals	Carbs	Fat	Protein
Subtotals				

Cals	Carbs	Fat	Protein

Weight

Notes / Excercise

Date _____   Su   Mo   Tu   We   Th   Fr   Sa

Meal 1   **Time:**

Food / Beverage	Cals	Carbs	Fat	Protein
Subtotals				

Meal 2   **Time:**

Food / Beverage	Cals	Carbs	Fat	Protein
Subtotals				

Meal 3   **Time:**

Food / Beverage	Cals	Carbs	Fat	Protein
Subtotals				

8 oz. servings of water ☐ ☐ ☐ ☐ ☐ ☐ ☐ ☐

Meal 4   Time:

Food / Beverage	Cals	Carbs	Fat	Protein
Subtotals				

Meal 5   Time:

Food / Beverage	Cals	Carbs	Fat	Protein
Subtotals				

Cals	Carbs	Fat	Protein		Weight

Notes / Excercise

Date _____   Su   Mo   Tu   We   Th   Fr   Sa

Meal 1   **Time:**

Food / Beverage	Cals	Carbs	Fat	Protein
Subtotals				

Meal 2   **Time:**

Food / Beverage	Cals	Carbs	Fat	Protein
Subtotals				

Meal 3   **Time:**

Food / Beverage	Cals	Carbs	Fat	Protein
Subtotals				

8 oz. servings of water ☐ ☐ ☐ ☐ ☐ ☐ ☐ ☐

Meal 4   Time:

Food / Beverage	Cals	Carbs	Fat	Protein
Subtotals				

Meal 5   Time:

Food / Beverage	Cals	Carbs	Fat	Protein
Subtotals				

Cals	Carbs	Fat	Protein

Weight

Notes / Excercise

_____

_____

_____

Date _____   Su   Mo   Tu   We   Th   Fr   Sa

Meal 1   **Time:**

Food / Beverage	Cals	Carbs	Fat	Protein
Subtotals				

Meal 2   **Time:**

Food / Beverage	Cals	Carbs	Fat	Protein
Subtotals				

Meal 3   **Time:**

Food / Beverage	Cals	Carbs	Fat	Protein
Subtotals				

8 oz. servings of water ☐ ☐ ☐ ☐ ☐ ☐ ☐ ☐

Meal 4   Time:

Food / Beverage	Cals	Carbs	Fat	Protein
Subtotals				

Meal 5   Time:

Food / Beverage	Cals	Carbs	Fat	Protein
Subtotals				

Cals	Carbs	Fat	Protein

Weight

Notes / Excercise

_____

_____

_____

Date _____   Su   Mo   Tu   We   Th   Fr   Sa

Meal 1   **Time:**

Food / Beverage	Cals	Carbs	Fat	Protein
Subtotals				

Meal 2   **Time:**

Food / Beverage	Cals	Carbs	Fat	Protein
Subtotals				

Meal 3   **Time:**

Food / Beverage	Cals	Carbs	Fat	Protein
Subtotals				

8 oz. servings of water ☐ ☐ ☐ ☐ ☐ ☐ ☐ ☐

Meal 4   Time:

Food / Beverage	Cals	Carbs	Fat	Protein
Subtotals				

Meal 5   Time:

Food / Beverage	Cals	Carbs	Fat	Protein
Subtotals				

Cals	Carbs	Fat	Protein

Weight

Notes / Excercise

_____

_____

_____

Date _____   Su   Mo   Tu   We   Th   Fr   Sa

Meal 1   **Time:**

Food / Beverage	Cals	Carbs	Fat	Protein
Subtotals				

Meal 2   **Time:**

Food / Beverage	Cals	Carbs	Fat	Protein
Subtotals				

Meal 3   **Time:**

Food / Beverage	Cals	Carbs	Fat	Protein
Subtotals				

8 oz. servings of water ☐ ☐ ☐ ☐ ☐ ☐ ☐ ☐

Meal 4   Time:

Food / Beverage	Cals	Carbs	Fat	Protein
Subtotals				

Meal 5   Time:

Food / Beverage	Cals	Carbs	Fat	Protein
Subtotals				

Cals	Carbs	Fat	Protein

Weight

Notes / Excercise

Date _____   Su   Mo   Tu   We   Th   Fr   Sa

Meal 1   Time:

Food / Beverage	Cals	Carbs	Fat	Protein
Subtotals				

Meal 2   Time:

Food / Beverage	Cals	Carbs	Fat	Protein
Subtotals				

Meal 3   Time:

Food / Beverage	Cals	Carbs	Fat	Protein
Subtotals				

8 oz. servings of water ☐ ☐ ☐ ☐ ☐ ☐ ☐ ☐

Meal 4   Time:

Food / Beverage	Cals	Carbs	Fat	Protein
Subtotals				

Meal 5   Time:

Food / Beverage	Cals	Carbs	Fat	Protein
Subtotals				

Cals	Carbs	Fat	Protein	Weight

Notes / Excercise
_____
_____
_____

Date _____   Su   Mo   Tu   We   Th   Fr   Sa

Meal 1   Time:

Food / Beverage	Cals	Carbs	Fat	Protein
Subtotals				

Meal 2   Time:

Food / Beverage	Cals	Carbs	Fat	Protein
Subtotals				

Meal 3   Time:

Food / Beverage	Cals	Carbs	Fat	Protein
Subtotals				

8 oz. servings of water ☐ ☐ ☐ ☐ ☐ ☐ ☐ ☐

Meal 4   Time:

Food / Beverage	Cals	Carbs	Fat	Protein
Subtotals				

Meal 5   Time:

Food / Beverage	Cals	Carbs	Fat	Protein
Subtotals				

Cals	Carbs	Fat	Protein

Weight

Notes / Excercise

Date _____   Su   Mo   Tu   We   Th   Fr   Sa

Meal 1   **Time:**

Food / Beverage	Cals	Carbs	Fat	Protein
Subtotals				

Meal 2   **Time:**

Food / Beverage	Cals	Carbs	Fat	Protein
Subtotals				

Meal 3   **Time:**

Food / Beverage	Cals	Carbs	Fat	Protein
Subtotals				

8 oz. servings of water ☐ ☐ ☐ ☐ ☐ ☐ ☐ ☐

Meal 4   **Time:**

Food / Beverage	Cals	Carbs	Fat	Protein
Subtotals				

Meal 5   **Time:**

Food / Beverage	Cals	Carbs	Fat	Protein
Subtotals				

Cals	Carbs	Fat	Protein

Weight

Notes / Excercise

Date _____   Su   Mo   Tu   We   Th   Fr   Sa

Meal 1   **Time:**

Food / Beverage	Cals	Carbs	Fat	Protein
Subtotals				

Meal 2   **Time:**

Food / Beverage	Cals	Carbs	Fat	Protein
Subtotals				

Meal 3   **Time:**

Food / Beverage	Cals	Carbs	Fat	Protein
Subtotals				

8 oz. servings of water ☐ ☐ ☐ ☐ ☐ ☐ ☐ ☐

Meal 4   Time:

Food / Beverage	Cals	Carbs	Fat	Protein
Subtotals				

Meal 5   Time:

Food / Beverage	Cals	Carbs	Fat	Protein
Subtotals				

Cals	Carbs	Fat	Protein	Weight

Notes / Excercise

Made in the USA
Coppell, TX
04 December 2021

67142425R00103